Headache Journal

```
     ┌─────────────────────────────────┐
     │      This journal belongs to    │
     │                                 │
     │   ............................. │
     │   ............................. │
     └─────────────────────────────────┘
```

Maintaining a headache journal helps you to identify the cause of your headache and what type it may be. It can help you identify trigger factors. It is especially useful in maintaining a food diary and spotting whether any particular food is triggering your headache.

How to use this journal:

- Note down the date, day of the week and time of starting and ending of the headache.

- Check the figures showing the different types of headaches. Tick the one which is similar to your own headache.

- Describe your diet in the hours before the headache occurred – it may indicate which food is a trigger factor for your headache.

- Tick off the number of glasses of water you had taken in the 6-8 hours prior to the headache. Dehydration is often a cause for cluster headaches or migraines.

- Note if you have any of the other listed trigger factors.

- List the medicines you are on. Also, mention which medicine gives you relief from the headache.

- Use the Notes section to mention any changes in your routine – stress, travelling, changes in medicine, very hot weather, humidity, depression etc.

Date: 24th November   Day of Week: Wednesday

| Time Occurred | | Time Ended | |

Type of Headache you have: Tick the right one:

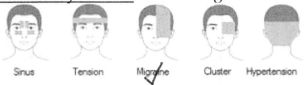

Sinus   Tension   Migraine ✓   Cluster   Hypertension

Severity on a Scale of 1-10 : Tick the right number:

| 1 | 2 | 3 | 4 | 5 | 6 | (7) | 8 | 9 | 10 |

Food Eaten During the Day:

Meal	Time	Food taken
Breakfast	11:00	Blueberries
Snacks	15:03	Popcorn
Lunch	14:00	rice noodles, corn, pepper, salt, basil, parsley, garlic
Tea		
Dinner		
Snacks		
Caffeine		
Alcohol		

How many glasses of water did you drink today:

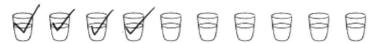

Other triggers: Tick which one affects you:

Stress ✓	Low blood Sugar	Eye Strain
Insomnia	PMS	Tiredness ✓
Dehydration	Motion Sickness	

Medicines taken daily:

Name	Dose	AM	PM

Notes:

Stress and tiredness from travelling

Date:..................... Day of Week:.......................

Time Occurred		Time Ended	

Type of Headache you have: Tick the right one:

Sinus Tension Migraine Cluster Hypertension

Severity on a Scale of 1-10 : Tick the right number:

1	2	3	4	5	6	7	8	9	10

Food Eaten During the Day:

Meal	Time	Food taken
Breakfast		
Snacks		
Lunch		
Tea		
Dinner		
Snacks		
Caffeine		
Alcohol		

How many glasses of water did you drink today:

🥛 🥛 🥛 🥛 🥛 🥛 🥛 🥛 🥛 🥛

Other triggers: Tick which one affects you:

Stress	Low blood Sugar	Eye Strain
Insomnia	PMS	Tiredness
Dehydration	Motion Sickness	

Medicines taken daily:

Name	Dose	AM	PM

Notes:
_____
_____
_____
_____
_____
_____
_____
_____
_____

Date:..................... Day of Week:.......................

Time Occurred		Time Ended	

Type of Headache you have: Tick the right one:

Sinus Tension Migraine Cluster Hypertension

Severity on a Scale of 1-10 : Tick the right number:

1	2	3	4	5	6	7	8	9	10

Food Eaten During the Day:

Meal	Time	Food taken
Breakfast		
Snacks		
Lunch		
Tea		
Dinner		
Snacks		
Caffeine		
Alcohol		

How many glasses of water did you drink today:

🥛 🥛 🥛 🥛 🥛 🥛 🥛 🥛 🥛 🥛

Other triggers: Tick which one affects you:

Stress	Low blood Sugar	Eye Strain
Insomnia	PMS	Tiredness
Dehydration	Motion Sickness	

Medicines taken daily:

Name	Dose	AM	PM

Notes:

_____
_____
_____
_____
_____
_____
_____
_____

Date:...................... Day of Week:........................

Time Occurred		Time Ended	

Type of Headache you have: Tick the right one:

Sinus	Tension	Migraine	Cluster	Hypertension

Severity on a Scale of 1-10 : Tick the right number:

1	2	3	4	5	6	7	8	9	10

Food Eaten During the Day:

Meal	Time	Food taken
Breakfast		
Snacks		
Lunch		
Tea		
Dinner		
Snacks		
Caffeine		
Alcohol		

How many glasses of water did you drink today:

Other triggers: Tick which one affects you:

Stress	Low blood Sugar	Eye Strain
Insomnia	PMS	Tiredness
Dehydration	Motion Sickness	

Medicines taken daily:

Name	Dose	AM	PM

Notes:
_____
_____
_____
_____
_____
_____
_____
_____
_____

Date:....................... Day of Week:........................

Time Occurred		Time Ended	

Type of Headache you have: Tick the right one:

Sinus   Tension   Migraine   Cluster   Hypertension

Severity on a Scale of 1-10 : Tick the right number:

1	2	3	4	5	6	7	8	9	10

Food Eaten During the Day:

Meal	Time	Food taken
Breakfast		
Snacks		
Lunch		
Tea		
Dinner		
Snacks		
Caffeine		
Alcohol		

How many glasses of water did you drink today:

🥛 🥛 🥛 🥛 🥛 🥛 🥛 🥛 🥛 🥛

Other triggers: Tick which one affects you:

Stress	Low blood Sugar	Eye Strain
Insomnia	PMS	Tiredness
Dehydration	Motion Sickness	

Medicines taken daily:

Name	Dose	AM	PM

Notes:

_____
_____
_____
_____
_____
_____
_____
_____

Date:...................... Day of Week:.........................

Time Occurred		Time Ended	

Type of Headache you have: Tick the right one:

Sinus Tension Migraine Cluster Hypertension

Severity on a Scale of 1-10 : Tick the right number:

1	2	3	4	5	6	7	8	9	10

Food Eaten During the Day:

Meal	Time	Food taken
Breakfast		
Snacks		
Lunch		
Tea		
Dinner		
Snacks		
Caffeine		
Alcohol		

How many glasses of water did you drink today:

🥛 🥛 🥛 🥛 🥛 🥛 🥛 🥛 🥛 🥛

Other triggers: Tick which one affects you:

Stress	Low blood Sugar	Eye Strain
Insomnia	PMS	Tiredness
Dehydration	Motion Sickness	

Medicines taken daily:

Name	Dose	AM	PM

Notes:

_____
_____
_____
_____
_____
_____
_____
_____
_____

Date:..................... Day of Week:......................

| Time Occurred | | Time Ended | |

Type of Headache you have: Tick the right one:

Sinus   Tension   Migraine   Cluster   Hypertension

Severity on a Scale of 1-10 : Tick the right number:

1	2	3	4	5	6	7	8	9	10

Food Eaten During the Day:

Meal	Time	Food taken
Breakfast		
Snacks		
Lunch		
Tea		
Dinner		
Snacks		
Caffeine		
Alcohol		

How many glasses of water did you drink today:

◻ ◻ ◻ ◻ ◻ ◻ ◻ ◻ ◻ ◻

Other triggers: Tick which one affects you:

Stress	Low blood Sugar	Eye Strain
Insomnia	PMS	Tiredness
Dehydration	Motion Sickness	

Medicines taken daily:

Name	Dose	AM	PM

Notes:

_____
_____
_____
_____
_____
_____
_____
_____

Date:………………… Day of Week:…………………..

Time Occurred		Time Ended	

Type of Headache you have: Tick the right one:

Sinus Tension Migraine Cluster Hypertension

Severity on a Scale of 1-10 : Tick the right number:

1	2	3	4	5	6	7	8	9	10

Food Eaten During the Day:

Meal	Time	Food taken
Breakfast		
Snacks		
Lunch		
Tea		
Dinner		
Snacks		
Caffeine		
Alcohol		

How many glasses of water did you drink today:

Other triggers: Tick which one affects you:

Stress	Low blood Sugar	Eye Strain
Insomnia	PMS	Tiredness
Dehydration	Motion Sickness	

Medicines taken daily:

Name	Dose	AM	PM

Notes:
_____
_____
_____
_____
_____
_____
_____
_____

Date:..................... Day of Week:......................

Time Occurred		Time Ended	

Type of Headache you have: Tick the right one:

Sinus   Tension   Migraine   Cluster   Hypertension

Severity on a Scale of 1-10 : Tick the right number:

1	2	3	4	5	6	7	8	9	10

Food Eaten During the Day:

Meal	Time	Food taken
Breakfast		
Snacks		
Lunch		
Tea		
Dinner		
Snacks		
Caffeine		
Alcohol		

How many glasses of water did you drink today:

🥛 🥛 🥛 🥛 🥛 🥛 🥛 🥛 🥛 🥛

Other triggers: Tick which one affects you:

Stress	Low blood Sugar	Eye Strain
Insomnia	PMS	Tiredness
Dehydration	Motion Sickness	

Medicines taken daily:

Name	Dose	AM	PM

Notes:

_____
_____
_____
_____
_____
_____
_____
_____

Date:......................   Day of Week:........................

Time Occurred		Time Ended	

Type of Headache you have: Tick the right one:

Sinus   Tension   Migraine   Cluster   Hypertension

Severity on a Scale of 1-10 : Tick the right number:

1	2	3	4	5	6	7	8	9	10

Food Eaten During the Day:

Meal	Time	Food taken
Breakfast		
Snacks		
Lunch		
Tea		
Dinner		
Snacks		
Caffeine		
Alcohol		

How many glasses of water did you drink today:

🥛 🥛 🥛 🥛 🥛 🥛 🥛 🥛 🥛 🥛

Other triggers: Tick which one affects you:

Stress	Low blood Sugar	Eye Strain
Insomnia	PMS	Tiredness
Dehydration	Motion Sickness	

Medicines taken daily:

Name	Dose	AM	PM

Notes:

_____
_____
_____
_____
_____
_____
_____
_____

Date:..................... Day of Week:......................

| Time Occurred | | Time Ended | |

Type of Headache you have: Tick the right one:

Sinus   Tension   Migraine   Cluster   Hypertension

Severity on a Scale of 1-10 : Tick the right number:

| 1 | 2 | 3 | 4 | 5 | 6 | 7 | 8 | 9 | 10 |

Food Eaten During the Day:

Meal	Time	Food taken
Breakfast		
Snacks		
Lunch		
Tea		
Dinner		
Snacks		
Caffeine		
Alcohol		

How many glasses of water did you drink today:

◻ ◻ ◻ ◻ ◻ ◻ ◻ ◻ ◻ ◻

Other triggers: Tick which one affects you:

Stress	Low blood Sugar	Eye Strain
Insomnia	PMS	Tiredness
Dehydration	Motion Sickness	

Medicines taken daily:

Name	Dose	AM	PM

Notes:

_____
_____
_____
_____
_____
_____
_____
_____

Date:..................... Day of Week:......................

Time Occurred		Time Ended	

Type of Headache you have: Tick the right one:

Sinus Tension Migraine Cluster Hypertension

Severity on a Scale of 1-10 : Tick the right number:

1	2	3	4	5	6	7	8	9	10

Food Eaten During the Day:

Meal	Time	Food taken
Breakfast		
Snacks		
Lunch		
Tea		
Dinner		
Snacks		
Caffeine		
Alcohol		

How many glasses of water did you drink today:

🥛 🥛 🥛 🥛 🥛 🥛 🥛 🥛 🥛 🥛

Other triggers: Tick which one affects you:

Stress	Low blood Sugar	Eye Strain
Insomnia	PMS	Tiredness
Dehydration	Motion Sickness	

Medicines taken daily:

Name	Dose	AM	PM

Notes:

_____
_____
_____
_____
_____
_____
_____
_____

Date:........................ Day of Week:........................

Time Occurred		Time Ended	

Type of Headache you have: Tick the right one:

Sinus Tension Migraine Cluster Hypertension

Severity on a Scale of 1-10 : Tick the right number:

1	2	3	4	5	6	7	8	9	10

Food Eaten During the Day:

Meal	Time	Food taken
Breakfast		
Snacks		
Lunch		
Tea		
Dinner		
Snacks		
Caffeine		
Alcohol		

How many glasses of water did you drink today:

Other triggers: Tick which one affects you:

Stress	Low blood Sugar	Eye Strain
Insomnia	PMS	Tiredness
Dehydration	Motion Sickness	

Medicines taken daily:

Name	Dose	AM	PM

Notes:

_____
_____
_____
_____
_____
_____
_____
_____

Date:......................   Day of Week:.......................

Time Occurred		Time Ended	

Type of Headache you have: Tick the right one:

Sinus   Tension   Migraine   Cluster   Hypertension

Severity on a Scale of 1-10 : Tick the right number:

1	2	3	4	5	6	7	8	9	10

Food Eaten During the Day:

Meal	Time	Food taken
Breakfast		
Snacks		
Lunch		
Tea		
Dinner		
Snacks		
Caffeine		
Alcohol		

How many glasses of water did you drink today:

🥛 🥛 🥛 🥛 🥛 🥛 🥛 🥛 🥛 🥛

Other triggers: Tick which one affects you:

Stress	Low blood Sugar	Eye Strain
Insomnia	PMS	Tiredness
Dehydration	Motion Sickness	

Medicines taken daily:

Name	Dose	AM	PM

Notes:

_____
_____
_____
_____
_____
_____
_____
_____

Date:…………………. Day of Week:…………………..

Time Occurred		Time Ended	

Type of Headache you have: Tick the right one:

Sinus   Tension   Migraine   Cluster   Hypertension

Severity on a Scale of 1-10 : Tick the right number:

1	2	3	4	5	6	7	8	9	10

Food Eaten During the Day:

Meal	Time	Food taken
Breakfast		
Snacks		
Lunch		
Tea		
Dinner		
Snacks		
Caffeine		
Alcohol		

How many glasses of water did you drink today:

Other triggers: Tick which one affects you:

Stress	Low blood Sugar	Eye Strain
Insomnia	PMS	Tiredness
Dehydration	Motion Sickness	

Medicines taken daily:

Name	Dose	AM	PM

Notes:
_____
_____
_____
_____
_____
_____
_____
_____

Date:…………………..   Day of Week:…………………..

Time Occurred		Time Ended	

Type of Headache you have: Tick the right one:

Sinus   Tension   Migraine   Cluster   Hypertension

Severity on a Scale of 1-10 : Tick the right number:

1	2	3	4	5	6	7	8	9	10

Food Eaten During the Day:

Meal	Time	Food taken
Breakfast		
Snacks		
Lunch		
Tea		
Dinner		
Snacks		
Caffeine		
Alcohol		

How many glasses of water did you drink today:

☐ ☐ ☐ ☐ ☐ ☐ ☐ ☐ ☐ ☐

Other triggers: Tick which one affects you:

Stress	Low blood Sugar	Eye Strain
Insomnia	PMS	Tiredness
Dehydration	Motion Sickness	

Medicines taken daily:

Name	Dose	AM	PM

Notes:

_____
_____
_____
_____
_____
_____
_____
_____

Date:...................... Day of Week:.......................

Time Occurred		Time Ended	

Type of Headache you have: Tick the right one:

Sinus   Tension   Migraine   Cluster   Hypertension

Severity on a Scale of 1-10 : Tick the right number:

1	2	3	4	5	6	7	8	9	10

Food Eaten During the Day:

Meal	Time	Food taken
Breakfast		
Snacks		
Lunch		
Tea		
Dinner		
Snacks		
Caffeine		
Alcohol		

How many glasses of water did you drink today:

🥛 🥛 🥛 🥛 🥛 🥛 🥛 🥛 🥛 🥛

Other triggers: Tick which one affects you:

Stress	Low blood Sugar	Eye Strain
Insomnia	PMS	Tiredness
Dehydration	Motion Sickness	

Medicines taken daily:

Name	Dose	AM	PM

Notes:

_____
_____
_____
_____
_____
_____
_____
_____

Date:.................... Day of Week:......................

Time Occurred		Time Ended	

Type of Headache you have: Tick the right one:

Sinus   Tension   Migraine   Cluster   Hypertension

Severity on a Scale of 1-10 : Tick the right number:

1	2	3	4	5	6	7	8	9	10

Food Eaten During the Day:

Meal	Time	Food taken
Breakfast		
Snacks		
Lunch		
Tea		
Dinner		
Snacks		
Caffeine		
Alcohol		

How many glasses of water did you drink today:

◯ ◯ ◯ ◯ ◯ ◯ ◯ ◯ ◯ ◯

Other triggers: Tick which one affects you:

Stress	Low blood Sugar	Eye Strain
Insomnia	PMS	Tiredness
Dehydration	Motion Sickness	

Medicines taken daily:

Name	Dose	AM	PM

Notes:

_____
_____
_____
_____
_____
_____
_____
_____
_____

Date:…………………. Day of Week:…………………..

Time Occurred		Time Ended	

Type of Headache you have: Tick the right one:

Sinus   Tension   Migraine   Cluster   Hypertension

Severity on a Scale of 1-10 : Tick the right number:

1	2	3	4	5	6	7	8	9	10

Food Eaten During the Day:

Meal	Time	Food taken
Breakfast		
Snacks		
Lunch		
Tea		
Dinner		
Snacks		
Caffeine		
Alcohol		

How many glasses of water did you drink today:

◻ ◻ ◻ ◻ ◻ ◻ ◻ ◻ ◻ ◻

Other triggers: Tick which one affects you:

Stress	Low blood Sugar	Eye Strain
Insomnia	PMS	Tiredness
Dehydration	Motion Sickness	

Medicines taken daily:

Name	Dose	AM	PM

Notes:

_____
_____
_____
_____
_____
_____
_____
_____

Date:………………… Day of Week:…………………..

Time Occurred		Time Ended	

Type of Headache you have: Tick the right one:

Sinus   Tension   Migraine   Cluster   Hypertension

Severity on a Scale of 1-10 : Tick the right number:

1	2	3	4	5	6	7	8	9	10

Food Eaten During the Day:

Meal	Time	Food taken
Breakfast		
Snacks		
Lunch		
Tea		
Dinner		
Snacks		
Caffeine		
Alcohol		

How many glasses of water did you drink today:

🥛 🥛 🥛 🥛 🥛 🥛 🥛 🥛 🥛 🥛

Other triggers: Tick which one affects you:

Stress	Low blood Sugar	Eye Strain
Insomnia	PMS	Tiredness
Dehydration	Motion Sickness	

Medicines taken daily:

Name	Dose	AM	PM

Notes:

_____
_____
_____
_____
_____
_____
_____
_____

Date:………………….. Day of Week:…………………..

Time Occurred		Time Ended	

Type of Headache you have: Tick the right one:

Sinus   Tension   Migraine   Cluster   Hypertension

Severity on a Scale of 1-10 : Tick the right number:

1	2	3	4	5	6	7	8	9	10

Food Eaten During the Day:

Meal	Time	Food taken
Breakfast		
Snacks		
Lunch		
Tea		
Dinner		
Snacks		
Caffeine		
Alcohol		

How many glasses of water did you drink today:

☐ ☐ ☐ ☐ ☐ ☐ ☐ ☐ ☐ ☐

Other triggers: Tick which one affects you:

Stress	Low blood Sugar	Eye Strain
Insomnia	PMS	Tiredness
Dehydration	Motion Sickness	

Medicines taken daily:

Name	Dose	AM	PM

Notes:

_____
_____
_____
_____
_____
_____
_____
_____
_____

Date:..................... Day of Week:.......................

Time Occurred		Time Ended	

Type of Headache you have: Tick the right one:

Sinus   Tension   Migraine   Cluster   Hypertension

Severity on a Scale of 1-10 : Tick the right number:

1	2	3	4	5	6	7	8	9	10

Food Eaten During the Day:

Meal	Time	Food taken
Breakfast		
Snacks		
Lunch		
Tea		
Dinner		
Snacks		
Caffeine		
Alcohol		

How many glasses of water did you drink today:

◻ ◻ ◻ ◻ ◻ ◻ ◻ ◻ ◻ ◻

Other triggers: Tick which one affects you:

Stress	Low blood Sugar	Eye Strain
Insomnia	PMS	Tiredness
Dehydration	Motion Sickness	

Medicines taken daily:

Name	Dose	AM	PM

Notes:

_____
_____
_____
_____
_____
_____
_____
_____

Date:..................... Day of Week:.......................

Time Occurred		Time Ended	

Type of Headache you have: Tick the right one:

Sinus   Tension   Migraine   Cluster   Hypertension

Severity on a Scale of 1-10 : Tick the right number:

1	2	3	4	5	6	7	8	9	10

Food Eaten During the Day:

Meal	Time	Food taken
Breakfast		
Snacks		
Lunch		
Tea		
Dinner		
Snacks		
Caffeine		
Alcohol		

How many glasses of water did you drink today:

🥛 🥛 🥛 🥛 🥛 🥛 🥛 🥛 🥛 🥛

Other triggers: Tick which one affects you:

Stress	Low blood Sugar	Eye Strain
Insomnia	PMS	Tiredness
Dehydration	Motion Sickness	

Medicines taken daily:

Name	Dose	AM	PM

Notes:

_____
_____
_____
_____
_____
_____
_____
_____
_____

Date:………………….   Day of Week:…………………..

Time Occurred		Time Ended	

Type of Headache you have: Tick the right one:

Sinus   Tension   Migraine   Cluster   Hypertension

Severity on a Scale of 1-10 : Tick the right number:

1	2	3	4	5	6	7	8	9	10

Food Eaten During the Day:

Meal	Time	Food taken
Breakfast		
Snacks		
Lunch		
Tea		
Dinner		
Snacks		
Caffeine		
Alcohol		

How many glasses of water did you drink today:

Other triggers: Tick which one affects you:

Stress	Low blood Sugar	Eye Strain
Insomnia	PMS	Tiredness
Dehydration	Motion Sickness	

Medicines taken daily:

Name	Dose	AM	PM

Notes:
_____
_____
_____
_____
_____
_____
_____
_____

Date:..................... Day of Week:.......................

Time Occurred		Time Ended	

Type of Headache you have: Tick the right one:

Sinus Tension Migraine Cluster Hypertension

Severity on a Scale of 1-10 : Tick the right number:

1	2	3	4	5	6	7	8	9	10

Food Eaten During the Day:

Meal	Time	Food taken
Breakfast		
Snacks		
Lunch		
Tea		
Dinner		
Snacks		
Caffeine		
Alcohol		

How many glasses of water did you drink today:

🥛 🥛 🥛 🥛 🥛 🥛 🥛 🥛 🥛 🥛

Other triggers: Tick which one affects you:

Stress	Low blood Sugar	Eye Strain
Insomnia	PMS	Tiredness
Dehydration	Motion Sickness	

Medicines taken daily:

Name	Dose	AM	PM

Notes:

_____
_____
_____
_____
_____
_____
_____
_____

Date:...................... Day of Week:..........................

Time Occurred		Time Ended	

Type of Headache you have: Tick the right one:

Sinus Tension Migraine Cluster Hypertension

Severity on a Scale of 1-10 : Tick the right number:

1	2	3	4	5	6	7	8	9	10

Food Eaten During the Day:

Meal	Time	Food taken
Breakfast		
Snacks		
Lunch		
Tea		
Dinner		
Snacks		
Caffeine		
Alcohol		

How many glasses of water did you drink today:

Other triggers: Tick which one affects you:

Stress	Low blood Sugar	Eye Strain
Insomnia	PMS	Tiredness
Dehydration	Motion Sickness	

Medicines taken daily:

Name	Dose	AM	PM

Notes:
_____
_____
_____
_____
_____
_____
_____
_____

Date:..................... Day of Week:......................

Time Occurred		Time Ended	

Type of Headache you have: Tick the right one:

Sinus   Tension   Migraine   Cluster   Hypertension

Severity on a Scale of 1-10 : Tick the right number:

1	2	3	4	5	6	7	8	9	10

Food Eaten During the Day:

Meal	Time	Food taken
Breakfast		
Snacks		
Lunch		
Tea		
Dinner		
Snacks		
Caffeine		
Alcohol		

How many glasses of water did you drink today:

Other triggers: Tick which one affects you:

Stress	Low blood Sugar	Eye Strain
Insomnia	PMS	Tiredness
Dehydration	Motion Sickness	

Medicines taken daily:

Name	Dose	AM	PM

Notes:
_____
_____
_____
_____
_____
_____
_____
_____

Date:..................... Day of Week:.......................

Time Occurred		Time Ended	

Type of Headache you have: Tick the right one:

Sinus   Tension   Migraine   Cluster   Hypertension

Severity on a Scale of 1-10 : Tick the right number:

1	2	3	4	5	6	7	8	9	10

Food Eaten During the Day:

Meal	Time	Food taken
Breakfast		
Snacks		
Lunch		
Tea		
Dinner		
Snacks		
Caffeine		
Alcohol		

How many glasses of water did you drink today:

🥛 🥛 🥛 🥛 🥛 🥛 🥛 🥛 🥛 🥛

Other triggers: Tick which one affects you:

Stress	Low blood Sugar	Eye Strain
Insomnia	PMS	Tiredness
Dehydration	Motion Sickness	

Medicines taken daily:

Name	Dose	AM	PM

Notes:

_____
_____
_____
_____
_____
_____
_____
_____

Date:…………………. Day of Week:…………………..

Time Occurred		Time Ended	

Type of Headache you have: Tick the right one:

Sinus   Tension   Migraine   Cluster   Hypertension

Severity on a Scale of 1-10 : Tick the right number:

1	2	3	4	5	6	7	8	9	10

Food Eaten During the Day:

Meal	Time	Food taken
Breakfast		
Snacks		
Lunch		
Tea		
Dinner		
Snacks		
Caffeine		
Alcohol		

How many glasses of water did you drink today:

🥛 🥛 🥛 🥛 🥛 🥛 🥛 🥛 🥛 🥛

Other triggers: Tick which one affects you:

Stress	Low blood Sugar	Eye Strain
Insomnia	PMS	Tiredness
Dehydration	Motion Sickness	

Medicines taken daily:

Name	Dose	AM	PM

Notes:

_____
_____
_____
_____
_____
_____
_____
_____
_____

Date:…………………. Day of Week:…………………..

Time Occurred		Time Ended	

Type of Headache you have: Tick the right one:

Sinus Tension Migraine Cluster Hypertension

Severity on a Scale of 1-10 : Tick the right number:

1	2	3	4	5	6	7	8	9	10

Food Eaten During the Day:

Meal	Time	Food taken
Breakfast		
Snacks		
Lunch		
Tea		
Dinner		
Snacks		
Caffeine		
Alcohol		

How many glasses of water did you drink today:

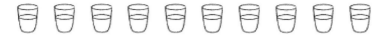

Other triggers: Tick which one affects you:

Stress	Low blood Sugar	Eye Strain
Insomnia	PMS	Tiredness
Dehydration	Motion Sickness	

Medicines taken daily:

Name	Dose	AM	PM

Notes:

_____
_____
_____
_____
_____
_____
_____
_____

Date:..................... Day of Week:.......................

Time Occurred		Time Ended	

Type of Headache you have: Tick the right one:

Sinus Tension Migraine Cluster Hypertension

Severity on a Scale of 1-10 : Tick the right number:

1	2	3	4	5	6	7	8	9	10

Food Eaten During the Day:

Meal	Time	Food taken
Breakfast		
Snacks		
Lunch		
Tea		
Dinner		
Snacks		
Caffeine		
Alcohol		

How many glasses of water did you drink today:

🥛 🥛 🥛 🥛 🥛 🥛 🥛 🥛 🥛 🥛

Other triggers: Tick which one affects you:

Stress	Low blood Sugar	Eye Strain
Insomnia	PMS	Tiredness
Dehydration	Motion Sickness	

Medicines taken daily:

Name	Dose	AM	PM

Notes:

_____
_____
_____
_____
_____
_____
_____
_____

Date:.................... Day of Week:........................

Time Occurred		Time Ended	

Type of Headache you have: Tick the right one:

Sinus Tension Migraine Cluster Hypertension

Severity on a Scale of 1-10 : Tick the right number:

1	2	3	4	5	6	7	8	9	10

Food Eaten During the Day:

Meal	Time	Food taken
Breakfast		
Snacks		
Lunch		
Tea		
Dinner		
Snacks		
Caffeine		
Alcohol		

How many glasses of water did you drink today:

🥛 🥛 🥛 🥛 🥛 🥛 🥛 🥛 🥛 🥛

Other triggers: Tick which one affects you:

Stress	Low blood Sugar	Eye Strain
Insomnia	PMS	Tiredness
Dehydration	Motion Sickness	

Medicines taken daily:

Name	Dose	AM	PM

Notes:

_____
_____
_____
_____
_____
_____
_____
_____
_____

Date:..................... Day of Week:.......................

Time Occurred		Time Ended	

Type of Headache you have: Tick the right one:

Sinus   Tension   Migraine   Cluster   Hypertension

Severity on a Scale of 1-10 : Tick the right number:

1	2	3	4	5	6	7	8	9	10

Food Eaten During the Day:

Meal	Time	Food taken
Breakfast		
Snacks		
Lunch		
Tea		
Dinner		
Snacks		
Caffeine		
Alcohol		

How many glasses of water did you drink today:

◻ ◻ ◻ ◻ ◻ ◻ ◻ ◻ ◻ ◻

Other triggers: Tick which one affects you:

Stress	Low blood Sugar	Eye Strain
Insomnia	PMS	Tiredness
Dehydration	Motion Sickness	

Medicines taken daily:

Name	Dose	AM	PM

Notes:

_____
_____
_____
_____
_____
_____
_____
_____

Date:........................ Day of Week:..........................

Time Occurred		Time Ended	

Type of Headache you have: Tick the right one:

Sinus   Tension   Migraine   Cluster   Hypertension

Severity on a Scale of 1-10 : Tick the right number:

1	2	3	4	5	6	7	8	9	10

Food Eaten During the Day:

Meal	Time	Food taken
Breakfast		
Snacks		
Lunch		
Tea		
Dinner		
Snacks		
Caffeine		
Alcohol		

How many glasses of water did you drink today:

🥛 🥛 🥛 🥛 🥛 🥛 🥛 🥛 🥛 🥛

Other triggers: Tick which one affects you:

Stress	Low blood Sugar	Eye Strain
Insomnia	PMS	Tiredness
Dehydration	Motion Sickness	

Medicines taken daily:

Name	Dose	AM	PM

Notes:

_____
_____
_____
_____
_____
_____
_____
_____
_____

Date:..................... Day of Week:......................

Time Occurred		Time Ended	

Type of Headache you have: Tick the right one:

Sinus   Tension   Migraine   Cluster   Hypertension

Severity on a Scale of 1-10 : Tick the right number:

1	2	3	4	5	6	7	8	9	10

Food Eaten During the Day:

Meal	Time	Food taken
Breakfast		
Snacks		
Lunch		
Tea		
Dinner		
Snacks		
Caffeine		
Alcohol		

How many glasses of water did you drink today:

Other triggers: Tick which one affects you:

Stress	Low blood Sugar	Eye Strain
Insomnia	PMS	Tiredness
Dehydration	Motion Sickness	

Medicines taken daily:

Name	Dose	AM	PM

Notes:
_____
_____
_____
_____
_____
_____
_____
_____

Date:...................... Day of Week:.......................

Time Occurred		Time Ended	

Type of Headache you have: Tick the right one:

Sinus Tension Migraine Cluster Hypertension

Severity on a Scale of 1-10 : Tick the right number:

1	2	3	4	5	6	7	8	9	10

Food Eaten During the Day:

Meal	Time	Food taken
Breakfast		
Snacks		
Lunch		
Tea		
Dinner		
Snacks		
Caffeine		
Alcohol		

How many glasses of water did you drink today:

☐ ☐ ☐ ☐ ☐ ☐ ☐ ☐ ☐ ☐

Other triggers: Tick which one affects you:

Stress	Low blood Sugar	Eye Strain
Insomnia	PMS	Tiredness
Dehydration	Motion Sickness	

Medicines taken daily:

Name	Dose	AM	PM

Notes:

_____
_____
_____
_____
_____
_____
_____
_____

Date:………………….   Day of Week:…………………..

| Time Occurred | | Time Ended | |

Type of Headache you have: Tick the right one:

Sinus   Tension   Migraine   Cluster   Hypertension

Severity on a Scale of 1-10 : Tick the right number:

| 1 | 2 | 3 | 4 | 5 | 6 | 7 | 8 | 9 | 10 |

Food Eaten During the Day:

Meal	Time	Food taken
Breakfast		
Snacks		
Lunch		
Tea		
Dinner		
Snacks		
Caffeine		
Alcohol		

How many glasses of water did you drink today:

◻ ◻ ◻ ◻ ◻ ◻ ◻ ◻ ◻ ◻

Other triggers: Tick which one affects you:

Stress	Low blood Sugar	Eye Strain
Insomnia	PMS	Tiredness
Dehydration	Motion Sickness	

Medicines taken daily:

Name	Dose	AM	PM

Notes:

_____
_____
_____
_____
_____
_____
_____
_____

Date:..................... Day of Week:........................

Time Occurred		Time Ended	

Type of Headache you have: Tick the right one:

Sinus   Tension   Migraine   Cluster   Hypertension

Severity on a Scale of 1-10 : Tick the right number:

1	2	3	4	5	6	7	8	9	10

Food Eaten During the Day:

Meal	Time	Food taken
Breakfast		
Snacks		
Lunch		
Tea		
Dinner		
Snacks		
Caffeine		
Alcohol		

How many glasses of water did you drink today:

☐ ☐ ☐ ☐ ☐ ☐ ☐ ☐ ☐ ☐

Other triggers: Tick which one affects you:

Stress	Low blood Sugar	Eye Strain
Insomnia	PMS	Tiredness
Dehydration	Motion Sickness	

Medicines taken daily:

Name	Dose	AM	PM

Notes:

_____
_____
_____
_____
_____
_____
_____
_____

Date:..................... Day of Week:.......................

Time Occurred		Time Ended	

Type of Headache you have: Tick the right one:

Sinus   Tension   Migraine   Cluster   Hypertension

Severity on a Scale of 1-10 : Tick the right number:

1	2	3	4	5	6	7	8	9	10

Food Eaten During the Day:

Meal	Time	Food taken
Breakfast		
Snacks		
Lunch		
Tea		
Dinner		
Snacks		
Caffeine		
Alcohol		

How many glasses of water did you drink today:

Other triggers: Tick which one affects you:

Stress	Low blood Sugar	Eye Strain
Insomnia	PMS	Tiredness
Dehydration	Motion Sickness	

Medicines taken daily:

Name	Dose	AM	PM

Notes:

_____
_____
_____
_____
_____
_____
_____
_____
_____

Date:………………….   Day of Week:…………………..

Time Occurred		Time Ended	

Type of Headache you have: Tick the right one:

Sinus   Tension   Migraine   Cluster   Hypertension

Severity on a Scale of 1-10 : Tick the right number:

1	2	3	4	5	6	7	8	9	10

Food Eaten During the Day:

Meal	Time	Food taken
Breakfast		
Snacks		
Lunch		
Tea		
Dinner		
Snacks		
Caffeine		
Alcohol		

How many glasses of water did you drink today:

🥛 🥛 🥛 🥛 🥛 🥛 🥛 🥛 🥛 🥛

Other triggers: Tick which one affects you:

Stress	Low blood Sugar	Eye Strain
Insomnia	PMS	Tiredness
Dehydration	Motion Sickness	

Medicines taken daily:

Name	Dose	AM	PM

Notes:

_____
_____
_____
_____
_____
_____
_____
_____
_____

Date:.......................   Day of Week:..........................

Time Occurred		Time Ended	

Type of Headache you have: Tick the right one:

Sinus   Tension   Migraine   Cluster   Hypertension

Severity on a Scale of 1-10 : Tick the right number:

1	2	3	4	5	6	7	8	9	10

Food Eaten During the Day:

Meal	Time	Food taken
Breakfast		
Snacks		
Lunch		
Tea		
Dinner		
Snacks		
Caffeine		
Alcohol		

How many glasses of water did you drink today:

🥛 🥛 🥛 🥛 🥛 🥛 🥛 🥛 🥛 🥛

Other triggers: Tick which one affects you:

Stress	Low blood Sugar	Eye Strain
Insomnia	PMS	Tiredness
Dehydration	Motion Sickness	

Medicines taken daily:

Name	Dose	AM	PM

Notes:

_____
_____
_____
_____
_____
_____
_____
_____
_____

Date:………………….   Day of Week:…………………..

Time Occurred		Time Ended	

Type of Headache you have: Tick the right one:

Sinus   Tension   Migraine   Cluster   Hypertension

Severity on a Scale of 1-10 : Tick the right number:

1	2	3	4	5	6	7	8	9	10

Food Eaten During the Day:

Meal	Time	Food taken
Breakfast		
Snacks		
Lunch		
Tea		
Dinner		
Snacks		
Caffeine		
Alcohol		

How many glasses of water did you drink today:

◯ ◯ ◯ ◯ ◯ ◯ ◯ ◯ ◯ ◯

Other triggers: Tick which one affects you:

Stress	Low blood Sugar	Eye Strain
Insomnia	PMS	Tiredness
Dehydration	Motion Sickness	

Medicines taken daily:

Name	Dose	AM	PM

Notes:

_____
_____
_____
_____
_____
_____
_____
_____

Date:..................... Day of Week:.......................

Time Occurred		Time Ended	

Type of Headache you have: Tick the right one:

Sinus Tension Migraine Cluster Hypertension

Severity on a Scale of 1-10 : Tick the right number:

1	2	3	4	5	6	7	8	9	10

Food Eaten During the Day:

Meal	Time	Food taken
Breakfast		
Snacks		
Lunch		
Tea		
Dinner		
Snacks		
Caffeine		
Alcohol		

How many glasses of water did you drink today:

☐ ☐ ☐ ☐ ☐ ☐ ☐ ☐ ☐ ☐

Other triggers: Tick which one affects you:

Stress	Low blood Sugar	Eye Strain
Insomnia	PMS	Tiredness
Dehydration	Motion Sickness	

Medicines taken daily:

Name	Dose	AM	PM

Notes:

_____
_____
_____
_____
_____
_____
_____
_____

Date:....................... Day of Week:........................

Time Occurred		Time Ended	

Type of Headache you have: Tick the right one:

Sinus Tension Migraine Cluster Hypertension

Severity on a Scale of 1-10 : Tick the right number:

1	2	3	4	5	6	7	8	9	10

Food Eaten During the Day:

Meal	Time	Food taken
Breakfast		
Snacks		
Lunch		
Tea		
Dinner		
Snacks		
Caffeine		
Alcohol		

How many glasses of water did you drink today:

◻ ◻ ◻ ◻ ◻ ◻ ◻ ◻ ◻ ◻

Other triggers: Tick which one affects you:

Stress	Low blood Sugar	Eye Strain
Insomnia	PMS	Tiredness
Dehydration	Motion Sickness	

Medicines taken daily:

Name	Dose	AM	PM

Notes:

_____
_____
_____
_____
_____
_____
_____
_____

Date:..................... Day of Week:.......................

Time Occurred		Time Ended	

Type of Headache you have: Tick the right one:

Sinus Tension Migraine Cluster Hypertension

Severity on a Scale of 1-10 : Tick the right number:

1	2	3	4	5	6	7	8	9	10

Food Eaten During the Day:

Meal	Time	Food taken
Breakfast		
Snacks		
Lunch		
Tea		
Dinner		
Snacks		
Caffeine		
Alcohol		

How many glasses of water did you drink today:

🥛 🥛 🥛 🥛 🥛 🥛 🥛 🥛 🥛 🥛

Other triggers: Tick which one affects you:

Stress	Low blood Sugar	Eye Strain
Insomnia	PMS	Tiredness
Dehydration	Motion Sickness	

Medicines taken daily:

Name	Dose	AM	PM

Notes:

_____
_____
_____
_____
_____
_____
_____
_____

Date:…………………. Day of Week:…………………..

Time Occurred		Time Ended	

Type of Headache you have: Tick the right one:

Sinus	Tension	Migraine	Cluster	Hypertension

Severity on a Scale of 1-10 : Tick the right number:

1	2	3	4	5	6	7	8	9	10

Food Eaten During the Day:

Meal	Time	Food taken
Breakfast		
Snacks		
Lunch		
Tea		
Dinner		
Snacks		
Caffeine		
Alcohol		

How many glasses of water did you drink today:

🥛 🥛 🥛 🥛 🥛 🥛 🥛 🥛 🥛 🥛

Other triggers: Tick which one affects you:

Stress	Low blood Sugar	Eye Strain
Insomnia	PMS	Tiredness
Dehydration	Motion Sickness	

Medicines taken daily:

Name	Dose	AM	PM

Notes:

_____
_____
_____
_____
_____
_____
_____
_____

Date:..................... Day of Week:......................

Time Occurred		Time Ended	

Type of Headache you have: Tick the right one:

Sinus   Tension   Migraine   Cluster   Hypertension

Severity on a Scale of 1-10 : Tick the right number:

1	2	3	4	5	6	7	8	9	10

Food Eaten During the Day:

Meal	Time	Food taken
Breakfast		
Snacks		
Lunch		
Tea		
Dinner		
Snacks		
Caffeine		
Alcohol		

How many glasses of water did you drink today:

⊔ ⊔ ⊔ ⊔ ⊔ ⊔ ⊔ ⊔ ⊔ ⊔

Other triggers: Tick which one affects you:

Stress	Low blood Sugar	Eye Strain
Insomnia	PMS	Tiredness
Dehydration	Motion Sickness	

Medicines taken daily:

Name	Dose	AM	PM

Notes:

_____
_____
_____
_____
_____
_____
_____
_____

Date:……………….   Day of Week:………………..

Time Occurred		Time Ended	

Type of Headache you have: Tick the right one:

Sinus   Tension   Migraine   Cluster   Hypertension

Severity on a Scale of 1-10 : Tick the right number:

1	2	3	4	5	6	7	8	9	10

Food Eaten During the Day:

Meal	Time	Food taken
Breakfast		
Snacks		
Lunch		
Tea		
Dinner		
Snacks		
Caffeine		
Alcohol		

How many glasses of water did you drink today:

☐ ☐ ☐ ☐ ☐ ☐ ☐ ☐ ☐ ☐

Other triggers: Tick which one affects you:

Stress	Low blood Sugar	Eye Strain
Insomnia	PMS	Tiredness
Dehydration	Motion Sickness	

Medicines taken daily:

Name	Dose	AM	PM

Notes:

_____
_____
_____
_____
_____
_____
_____
_____
_____

Date:………………….   Day of Week:…………………..

| Time Occurred | | Time Ended | |

Type of Headache you have: Tick the right one:

Sinus   Tension   Migraine   Cluster   Hypertension

Severity on a Scale of 1-10 : Tick the right number:

| 1 | 2 | 3 | 4 | 5 | 6 | 7 | 8 | 9 | 10 |

Food Eaten During the Day:

Meal	Time	Food taken
Breakfast		
Snacks		
Lunch		
Tea		
Dinner		
Snacks		
Caffeine		
Alcohol		

How many glasses of water did you drink today:

Other triggers: Tick which one affects you:

Stress	Low blood Sugar	Eye Strain
Insomnia	PMS	Tiredness
Dehydration	Motion Sickness	

Medicines taken daily:

Name	Dose	AM	PM

Notes:

_____
_____
_____
_____
_____
_____
_____
_____

Date:……………….   Day of Week:…………………..

Time Occurred		Time Ended	

Type of Headache you have: Tick the right one:

Sinus   Tension   Migraine   Cluster   Hypertension

Severity on a Scale of 1-10 : Tick the right number:

1	2	3	4	5	6	7	8	9	10

Food Eaten During the Day:

Meal	Time	Food taken
Breakfast		
Snacks		
Lunch		
Tea		
Dinner		
Snacks		
Caffeine		
Alcohol		

How many glasses of water did you drink today:

◯ ◯ ◯ ◯ ◯ ◯ ◯ ◯ ◯ ◯

Other triggers: Tick which one affects you:

Stress	Low blood Sugar	Eye Strain
Insomnia	PMS	Tiredness
Dehydration	Motion Sickness	

Medicines taken daily:

Name	Dose	AM	PM

Notes:

_____
_____
_____
_____
_____
_____
_____
_____
_____

Date:………………….   Day of Week:…………………..

| Time Occurred | | Time Ended | |

Type of Headache you have: Tick the right one:

Sinus   Tension   Migraine   Cluster   Hypertension

Severity on a Scale of 1-10 : Tick the right number:

| 1 | 2 | 3 | 4 | 5 | 6 | 7 | 8 | 9 | 10 |

Food Eaten During the Day:

Meal	Time	Food taken
Breakfast		
Snacks		
Lunch		
Tea		
Dinner		
Snacks		
Caffeine		
Alcohol		

How many glasses of water did you drink today:

Other triggers: Tick which one affects you:

Stress	Low blood Sugar	Eye Strain
Insomnia	PMS	Tiredness
Dehydration	Motion Sickness	

Medicines taken daily:

Name	Dose	AM	PM

Notes:

_____
_____
_____
_____
_____
_____
_____
_____
_____

Date:........................   Day of Week:..........................

Time Occurred		Time Ended	

Type of Headache you have: Tick the right one:

Sinus   Tension   Migraine   Cluster   Hypertension

Severity on a Scale of 1-10 : Tick the right number:

1	2	3	4	5	6	7	8	9	10

Food Eaten During the Day:

Meal	Time	Food taken
Breakfast		
Snacks		
Lunch		
Tea		
Dinner		
Snacks		
Caffeine		
Alcohol		

How many glasses of water did you drink today:

🥛 🥛 🥛 🥛 🥛 🥛 🥛 🥛 🥛 🥛

Other triggers: Tick which one affects you:

Stress	Low blood Sugar	Eye Strain
Insomnia	PMS	Tiredness
Dehydration	Motion Sickness	

Medicines taken daily:

Name	Dose	AM	PM

Notes:

_____
_____
_____
_____
_____
_____
_____
_____

Date:..................... Day of Week:.......................

Time Occurred		Time Ended	

Type of Headache you have: Tick the right one:

Sinus   Tension   Migraine   Cluster   Hypertension

Severity on a Scale of 1-10 : Tick the right number:

1	2	3	4	5	6	7	8	9	10

Food Eaten During the Day:

Meal	Time	Food taken
Breakfast		
Snacks		
Lunch		
Tea		
Dinner		
Snacks		
Caffeine		
Alcohol		

How many glasses of water did you drink today:

☐ ☐ ☐ ☐ ☐ ☐ ☐ ☐ ☐ ☐

Other triggers: Tick which one affects you:

Stress	Low blood Sugar	Eye Strain
Insomnia	PMS	Tiredness
Dehydration	Motion Sickness	

Medicines taken daily:

Name	Dose	AM	PM

Notes:

_____
_____
_____
_____
_____
_____
_____
_____

Date:..................... Day of Week:........................

Time Occurred		Time Ended	

Type of Headache you have: Tick the right one:

Sinus   Tension   Migraine   Cluster   Hypertension

Severity on a Scale of 1-10 : Tick the right number:

1	2	3	4	5	6	7	8	9	10

Food Eaten During the Day:

Meal	Time	Food taken
Breakfast		
Snacks		
Lunch		
Tea		
Dinner		
Snacks		
Caffeine		
Alcohol		

How many glasses of water did you drink today:

🥛 🥛 🥛 🥛 🥛 🥛 🥛 🥛 🥛 🥛

Other triggers: Tick which one affects you:

Stress	Low blood Sugar	Eye Strain
Insomnia	PMS	Tiredness
Dehydration	Motion Sickness	

Medicines taken daily:

Name	Dose	AM	PM

Notes:

_____
_____
_____
_____
_____
_____
_____
_____
_____

Date:..................... Day of Week:......................

Time Occurred		Time Ended	

Type of Headache you have: Tick the right one:

Sinus   Tension   Migraine   Cluster   Hypertension

Severity on a Scale of 1-10 : Tick the right number:

1	2	3	4	5	6	7	8	9	10

Food Eaten During the Day:

Meal	Time	Food taken
Breakfast		
Snacks		
Lunch		
Tea		
Dinner		
Snacks		
Caffeine		
Alcohol		

How many glasses of water did you drink today:

🥛 🥛 🥛 🥛 🥛 🥛 🥛 🥛 🥛 🥛

Other triggers: Tick which one affects you:

Stress	Low blood Sugar	Eye Strain
Insomnia	PMS	Tiredness
Dehydration	Motion Sickness	

Medicines taken daily:

Name	Dose	AM	PM

Notes:

_____
_____
_____
_____
_____
_____
_____
_____
_____

Date:..................... Day of Week:......................

Time Occurred		Time Ended	

Type of Headache you have: Tick the right one:

Sinus   Tension   Migraine   Cluster   Hypertension

Severity on a Scale of 1-10 : Tick the right number:

1	2	3	4	5	6	7	8	9	10

Food Eaten During the Day:

Meal	Time	Food taken
Breakfast		
Snacks		
Lunch		
Tea		
Dinner		
Snacks		
Caffeine		
Alcohol		

How many glasses of water did you drink today:

🥛 🥛 🥛 🥛 🥛 🥛 🥛 🥛 🥛 🥛

Other triggers: Tick which one affects you:

Stress	Low blood Sugar	Eye Strain
Insomnia	PMS	Tiredness
Dehydration	Motion Sickness	

Medicines taken daily:

Name	Dose	AM	PM

Notes:

_____
_____
_____
_____
_____
_____
_____
_____

Date:......................   Day of Week:.........................

Time Occurred		Time Ended	

Type of Headache you have: Tick the right one:

Sinus   Tension   Migraine   Cluster   Hypertension

Severity on a Scale of 1-10 : Tick the right number:

1	2	3	4	5	6	7	8	9	10

Food Eaten During the Day:

Meal	Time	Food taken
Breakfast		
Snacks		
Lunch		
Tea		
Dinner		
Snacks		
Caffeine		
Alcohol		

How many glasses of water did you drink today:

🥛 🥛 🥛 🥛 🥛 🥛 🥛 🥛 🥛 🥛

Other triggers: Tick which one affects you:

Stress	Low blood Sugar	Eye Strain
Insomnia	PMS	Tiredness
Dehydration	Motion Sickness	

Medicines taken daily:

Name	Dose	AM	PM

Notes:

_____
_____
_____
_____
_____
_____
_____
_____

Date:………………….. Day of Week:…………………..

Time Occurred		Time Ended	

Type of Headache you have: Tick the right one:

Sinus Tension Migraine Cluster Hypertension

Severity on a Scale of 1-10 : Tick the right number:

1	2	3	4	5	6	7	8	9	10

Food Eaten During the Day:

Meal	Time	Food taken
Breakfast		
Snacks		
Lunch		
Tea		
Dinner		
Snacks		
Caffeine		
Alcohol		

How many glasses of water did you drink today:

○ ○ ○ ○ ○ ○ ○ ○ ○ ○

Other triggers: Tick which one affects you:

Stress	Low blood Sugar	Eye Strain
Insomnia	PMS	Tiredness
Dehydration	Motion Sickness	

Medicines taken daily:

Name	Dose	AM	PM

Notes:

_____
_____
_____
_____
_____
_____
_____
_____

Date:..................... Day of Week:.....................

Time Occurred		Time Ended	

Type of Headache you have: Tick the right one:

| Sinus | Tension | Migraine | Cluster | Hypertension |

Severity on a Scale of 1-10 : Tick the right number:

1	2	3	4	5	6	7	8	9	10

Food Eaten During the Day:

Meal	Time	Food taken
Breakfast		
Snacks		
Lunch		
Tea		
Dinner		
Snacks		
Caffeine		
Alcohol		

How many glasses of water did you drink today:

🥛 🥛 🥛 🥛 🥛 🥛 🥛 🥛 🥛 🥛

Other triggers: Tick which one affects you:

Stress	Low blood Sugar	Eye Strain
Insomnia	PMS	Tiredness
Dehydration	Motion Sickness	

Medicines taken daily:

Name	Dose	AM	PM

Notes:

_____
_____
_____
_____
_____
_____
_____
_____

Date:………………… Day of Week:……………………..

Time Occurred		Time Ended	

Type of Headache you have: Tick the right one:

Sinus   Tension   Migraine   Cluster   Hypertension

Severity on a Scale of 1-10 : Tick the right number:

1	2	3	4	5	6	7	8	9	10

Food Eaten During the Day:

Meal	Time	Food taken
Breakfast		
Snacks		
Lunch		
Tea		
Dinner		
Snacks		
Caffeine		
Alcohol		

How many glasses of water did you drink today:

◯ ◯ ◯ ◯ ◯ ◯ ◯ ◯ ◯ ◯

Other triggers: Tick which one affects you:

Stress	Low blood Sugar	Eye Strain
Insomnia	PMS	Tiredness
Dehydration	Motion Sickness	

Medicines taken daily:

Name	Dose	AM	PM

Notes:

_____
_____
_____
_____
_____
_____
_____
_____

Date:…………………..   Day of Week:…………………..

Time Occurred		Time Ended	

Type of Headache you have: Tick the right one:

Sinus   Tension   Migraine   Cluster   Hypertension

Severity on a Scale of 1-10 : Tick the right number:

1	2	3	4	5	6	7	8	9	10

Food Eaten During the Day:

Meal	Time	Food taken
Breakfast		
Snacks		
Lunch		
Tea		
Dinner		
Snacks		
Caffeine		
Alcohol		

How many glasses of water did you drink today:

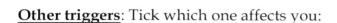

Other triggers: Tick which one affects you:

Stress	Low blood Sugar	Eye Strain
Insomnia	PMS	Tiredness
Dehydration	Motion Sickness	

Medicines taken daily:

Name	Dose	AM	PM

Notes:
_____
_____
_____
_____
_____
_____
_____
_____

7, 9, 10, 11, 12, 13, 17, 18, 20, 23, 25, 29

$$\frac{13 + 17}{2} = 15$$

29 − 6 = 23

25 − 7 = 18

23 − 18 = 5

28,000,000

28,750,085

28,705,185

Printed in Great Britain
by Amazon